<u>Drop Those Extra Pounds</u>

A Journey to a Lighter and Healthier You

BY

Kobus Fourie

DROP THOSE EXTRA POUNDS

First edition. April 29, 2023.

Copyright © 2023 Kobus Fourie.

ISBN: 979-8223372752

Written by Kobus Fourie.

Also by Kobus Fourie

Strange Facts and Wonders
20 Beddie Buy Stories For Kid's
Animals by the Alphabet
Stop That Bad Smoking Habit
Drop Those Extra Pounds
Lyric's For Everyone

Table of Contents

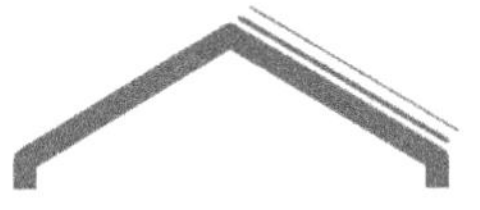

ACKNOWLEDGMENTS

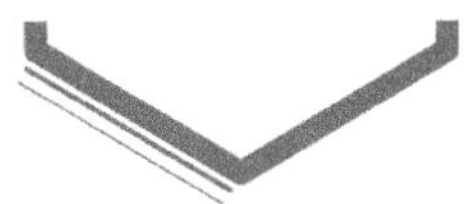

I would like to express my gratitude to the following individuals who have contributed to the creation of this weight loss book:

- My editor, who provided invaluable feedback and guidance throughout the writing process.
- The team of proofreaders who helped ensure the accuracy and clarity of the content.
- My family and friends who provided encouragement and support during the writing process.
- The healthcare professionals and nutritionists who provided their expert knowledge and advice.
- The individuals who generously shared their weight loss success stories and provided inspiration for this book.
- The readers who have chosen to embark on this weight loss journey and use this book as a resource to achieve their goals.

Thank you all for your contributions, encouragement, and support.

Sincerely,

Kobus Fourie

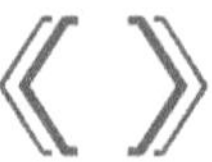

The writer is by no means an expert in weight loss or a health practitioner but thru personal experience are sharing what he learned

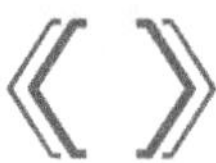

CHAPTER 1: UNDERSTANDING the basics of weight loss: calories in vs. calories out

Losing weight is a common goal for many people, but the process can often feel overwhelming and confusing. One of the most fundamental concepts to understand when it comes to weight loss is the balance between calories in and calories out. In this chapter, we will explore the basics of this concept and its implications for weight loss.

Calories in vs. calories out

At its core, weight loss is simply a matter of burning more calories than you consume. This balance between calories in and calories out is often referred to as energy balance. When you consume more calories than your body burns, you will gain weight. On the other hand, when you burn more calories than you consume, you will lose weight.

Calories in

Calories in refer to the calories you consume through food and beverages. It is important to note that not all calories are created equal. Different foods and drinks can have vastly different calorie contents, even if their serving sizes are similar. For example, a small serving of potato chips may contain several hundred calories, while a large serving of vegetables may contain only a fraction of that amount.

To effectively manage your calorie intake, it is important to be mindful of the types of foods and drinks you consume. High-calorie, high-fat, and high-sugar foods and beverages should be consumed in moderation, while low-calorie, nutrient-dense options such as fruits, vegetables, lean proteins, and whole grains should be prioritized.

Calories out

Calories out refer to the calories your body burns through physical activity and basic metabolic processes. Your body burns calories throughout the day, even when you are not engaging in formal exercise. This is known as your basal metabolic rate (BMR) and is influenced by factors such as your age, sex, weight, and muscle mass.

In addition to your BMR, you can also burn calories through physical activity. This can include structured exercise such as running, weightlifting, or yoga, as well as everyday activities such as walking, cleaning, and gardening. The more active you are, the more calories you will burn.

Understanding your calorie needs

To effectively manage your weight, it is important to have a good understanding of your individual calorie needs. This will help you to determine how many calories you should be consuming each day to maintain your current weight, as well as how many calories you should be consuming to reach your weight loss goals.

Your calorie needs are influenced by a variety of factors, including your age, sex, height, weight, and activity level. There are a variety of online calculators and tools that can help you to estimate your daily calorie needs based on these factors.

Creating a calorie deficit

To lose weight, you will need to create a calorie deficit, which means that you are consuming fewer calories than you are burning. There are a few different ways to achieve this, including:

1. Consuming fewer calories: By reducing your calorie intake, you can create a calorie deficit. This can be done by cutting back on high-calorie foods and beverages, reducing portion sizes, and making healthier food choices.
2. Increasing physical activity: By increasing your physical activity, you can burn more calories and create a calorie deficit. This can be done through structured exercise, such as going to the gym, as well as by incorporating more movement into your daily routine, such as taking the stairs instead of the elevator or going for a walk during your lunch break.
3. A combination of both: The most effective approach to weight loss is often a combination of reducing calorie intake and increasing physical activity. By doing both, you can create a larger calorie deficit and see results more quickly.

4 Monitoring progress

To ensure that you are on track to reaching your weight loss goals, it

Chapter 2: Creating a Personalized Meal Plan for Weight Loss

When it comes to losing weight, what you eat is just as important as how much you eat. A personalized meal plan can help you achieve your weight loss goals by ensuring that you're consuming the right balance of nutrients and calories.

Here are some steps to help you create a personalized meal plan for weight loss:

Step 1: Determine your daily calorie needs

The first step in creating a personalized meal plan for weight loss is to determine how many calories you need to consume each day. This can vary based on your age, gender, weight, height, and activity level.

There are many online calculators and mobile apps that can help you determine your daily calorie needs. Once you have this number, you can begin planning your meals and snacks accordingly.

Step 2: Set macronutrient goals

Macronutrients are the three major nutrients that our bodies need in large quantities: protein, carbohydrates, and fat. Each of these nutrients plays a unique role in the body, and getting the right balance of macronutrients can help you feel satisfied and energized throughout the day.

Protein: Protein is essential for building and repairing tissues, and it can also help you feel full and satisfied. Aim to consume lean sources of protein such as chicken, fish, beans, lentils, and tofu.

Carbohydrates: Carbohydrates provide energy for the body, but not all carbs are created equal. Choose complex carbohydrates such as whole grains, fruits, and vegetables, which provide fiber and nutrients in addition to energy.

Fat: Healthy fats such as those found in nuts, seeds, avocado, and olive oil can help you feel full and satisfied. However, it's important to keep portion sizes in mind, as fat is more calorie-dense than protein or carbs.

Step 3: Plan your meals and snacks

Once you have your daily calorie and macronutrient goals in mind, it's time to start planning your meals and snacks. Here are some tips to keep in mind:

- Include lean protein, complex carbohydrates, and healthy fats in each meal.
- Aim to fill half of your plate with non-starchy vegetables, such as leafy greens, broccoli, and peppers.
- Choose whole grains over refined grains, which can spike blood sugar levels and lead to overeating.
- Avoid sugary drinks and high-calorie snacks, such as chips and candy.
- Plan your meals and snacks in advance, so you're not tempted to reach for unhealthy options when you're hungry.

Step 4: Monitor your progress

It's important to monitor your progress as you follow your personalized meal plan for weight loss. Keep a food diary or use a mobile app to track your intake, and adjust your plan as needed if you're not seeing the results you want.

Remember, weight loss is not a one-size-fits-all approach. Your personalized meal plan should be tailored to your individual needs and preferences, and it should be sustainable in the long-term.

In addition to creating a personalized meal plan for weight loss, here are some additional tips to help you reach your goals:

- Stay hydrated by drinking plenty of water throughout the day.
- Aim to get at least 30 minutes of moderate-intensity exercise most days of the week.
- Get enough sleep each night, as lack of sleep can lead to overeating and weight gain.
- Practice stress-reducing techniques such as meditation or yoga to prevent emotional eating.

In conclusion, creating a personalized meal plan for weight loss can be a key component of achieving your weight loss goals. By determining your daily calorie needs, setting macronutrient goals, planning your meals and snacks, and monitoring your progress, you can create a sustainable plan that works for you. Remember to also incorporate

Chapter 3: Strategies for Meal Prep and Cooking Healthy Meals at Home

Meal prep and cooking healthy meals at home can be a game-changer when it comes to losing weight. By planning and preparing your meals in advance, you can ensure that you're making healthy choices and avoiding the temptation of less healthy options.

Here are some strategies for meal prep and cooking healthy meals at home:

1. Plan your meals in advance

Before you head to the grocery store, take some time to plan out your meals for the week. This will help you avoid impulse purchases and ensure that you have all the ingredients you need to make healthy meals.

Consider planning meals around lean sources of protein, whole grains, and non-starchy vegetables. You can also incorporate healthy fats such as avocado, nuts, and seeds.

1. Prep ingredients in advance

Once you've planned your meals, take some time to prep ingredients in advance. This can include washing and chopping vegetables, cooking whole grains, and marinating lean proteins.

By prepping ingredients in advance, you can save time during the week and make healthy meals more convenient.

1. Invest in quality kitchen tools

Having the right kitchen tools can make healthy meal prep and cooking a breeze. Consider investing in a good set of knives, a quality cutting board, and a food processor or blender.

Other helpful tools can include a slow cooker, instant pot, or air fryer, which can make meal prep and cooking more efficient.

1. Experiment with healthy recipes

Healthy eating doesn't have to be boring or bland. Experiment with new recipes that incorporate healthy ingredients and flavors.

You can find healthy recipes online, in cookbooks, or by asking friends and family for recommendations. Don't be afraid to try new things and get creative in the kitchen.

1. Portion out meals in advance

Portion control is an important part of healthy eating and weight loss. To make portion control easier, consider portioning out meals in advance.

You can use meal prep containers or resealable bags to portion out meals and snacks. This can help you avoid overeating and ensure that you're getting the right balance of nutrients.

1. Freeze meals for later

If you're short on time during the week, consider making larger batches of healthy meals and freezing them for later.

You can freeze meals in portioned containers or resealable bags for easy reheating. This can be a convenient way to ensure that you always have healthy meals on hand.

1. Make healthy swaps

When cooking at home, consider making healthy swaps to reduce calories and improve nutrition.

For example, you can use Greek yogurt instead of sour cream, swap out refined grains for whole grains, and use herbs and spices instead of salt for flavor.

In conclusion, meal prep and cooking healthy meals at home can be a key component of losing weight and improving overall health. By planning meals in advance, prepping ingredients, investing in quality kitchen tools, experimenting with healthy recipes, portioning out meals, freezing meals for later, and making healthy swaps, you can make healthy eating more convenient and enjoyable. Remember to also focus on balance and moderation, and don't be too hard on yourself if you slip up occasionally.

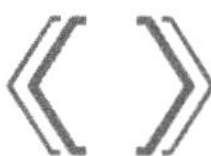

CHAPTER 4: THE ROLE of Protein, Carbohydrates, and Fats in Weight Loss

When it comes to weight loss, it's important to pay attention to the types of foods you're eating and the nutrients they contain. Protein, carbohydrates, and fats all play important roles in weight loss and overall health.

Protein

Protein is an essential nutrient that plays a crucial role in weight loss. It's important for building and repairing muscle, which can help increase metabolism and burn more calories.

Protein can also help you feel full and satisfied, which can prevent overeating and snacking between meals. In fact, studies have shown that increasing protein intake can lead to reduced calorie intake and weight loss.

Good sources of protein include lean meats, poultry, fish, eggs, beans, and lentils. You can also get protein from dairy products, such as Greek yogurt and cottage cheese, as well as plant-based sources, such as tofu and tempeh.

Carbohydrates

Carbohydrates are an important source of energy for the body, but not all carbohydrates are created equal when it comes to weight loss. Refined carbohydrates, such as white bread and sugary snacks, can lead to spikes in blood sugar and insulin levels, which can promote fat storage.

On the other hand, complex carbohydrates, such as whole grains, fruits, and vegetables, are high in fiber and nutrients and can help promote satiety and weight loss.

When choosing carbohydrates, aim for whole, minimally processed sources. Good options include brown rice, quinoa, sweet potatoes, berries, and leafy greens.

Fats

Fats are an important nutrient that plays many roles in the body, including providing energy and supporting cell growth and development. However, not all fats are created equal.

Trans fats and saturated fats, found in fried foods and high-fat animal products, can increase the risk of heart disease and weight gain. On the other hand, unsaturated fats, found in foods such as avocados, nuts, and fatty fish, can provide health benefits and promote weight loss.

When choosing fats, aim for healthy sources such as nuts, seeds, avocado, and fatty fish. Use oils such as olive oil, coconut oil, and canola oil in moderation.

Overall, a balanced diet that includes a variety of protein, carbohydrates, and healthy fats is key for weight loss and overall health. Aim to incorporate lean sources of protein, complex carbohydrates, and healthy fats into each meal and snack, and avoid highly processed and refined foods. Remember to also pay attention to portion sizes and aim for balance and moderation in your diet.

Chapter 5: Incorporating More Whole Foods and Plant-Based Foods into Your Diet

Incorporating more whole foods and plant-based foods into your diet is a great way to promote weight loss and overall health. Whole foods are minimally processed and contain a variety of nutrients, while plant-based foods are rich in fiber, vitamins, and minerals.

Here are some tips for incorporating more whole foods and plant-based foods into your diet:

1. Focus on fruits and vegetables: Aim to incorporate a variety of fruits and vegetables into each meal and snack. These foods are rich in fiber and nutrients and can help promote satiety and weight loss. Try to include a rainbow of colors, such as red peppers, green spinach, yellow squash, and purple berries.

2. Choose whole grains: Instead of refined grains, such as white bread and pasta, choose whole grains like brown rice, quinoa, and whole grain bread. These foods are high in fiber and can help promote satiety.

3. Incorporate legumes: Legumes, such as beans, lentils, and chickpeas, are great sources of plant-based protein and fiber. Try adding them to soups, salads, and stir-fries for a boost of nutrition.

4. Experiment with new recipes: There are many delicious and healthy recipes that incorporate whole foods and plant-based foods. Look for recipes online or in cookbooks and experiment with new ingredients and flavors.

5. Swap out processed snacks for whole food options:

Instead of reaching for chips or cookies, choose whole food snacks like nuts, fruit, or vegetable sticks with hummus.

6. Add herbs and spices for flavor: Instead of relying on high-calorie sauces and dressings, try adding herbs and spices for flavor. For example, try using fresh basil and oregano in pasta dishes instead of heavy sauces.

Incorporating more whole foods and plant-based foods into your diet can be a gradual process. Start by making small changes, such as adding a serving of vegetables to each meal, and gradually increasing your intake over time. Remember to also pay attention to portion sizes and aim for balance and moderation in your diet.

In addition to promoting weight loss, incorporating more whole foods and plant-based foods into your diet can have other health benefits, such as reducing the risk of chronic diseases like heart disease and type 2 diabetes. By focusing on whole, minimally processed foods and incorporating more plant-based options, you can improve your overall health and well-being.

Chapter 6: Keeping a Food Diary or Using a Food Tracking App to Monitor Your Intake

One of the most effective ways to lose weight is to keep track of what you're eating. By monitoring your food intake, you can become more aware of your eating habits and make changes to promote weight loss.

There are two main methods for tracking your food intake: keeping a food diary or using a food tracking app.

Keeping a Food Diary

Keeping a food diary involves writing down everything you eat and drink throughout the day. This can help you become more aware of your eating habits and identify areas where you can make changes to promote weight loss.

To keep a food diary, you can use a notebook or journal, or even a smartphone app. Be sure to record the type of food, portion size, and time of day that you ate. You can also include notes about how you felt before and after eating, such as hunger or satisfaction.

Using a Food Tracking App

Food tracking apps are another popular way to monitor your food intake. These apps allow you to log your meals and snacks and track your calorie intake, macronutrients, and micronutrients.

Some popular food tracking apps include MyFitnessPal, Lose It!, and Cronometer. These apps allow you to search for foods and drinks and log them quickly and easily. You can also set goals for calorie intake and macronutrient ratios, and the app will track your progress throughout the day.

Benefits of Tracking Your Food Intake

Tracking your food intake can have many benefits for weight loss and overall health. Here are some of the main benefits:

1. Increased awareness: By tracking your food intake, you become more aware of what you're eating and drinking throughout the day. This can help you identify areas where you can make changes to promote weight loss.

2. Accountability: Tracking your food intake can also help you stay accountable to your weight loss goals. When you see what you're eating on a daily basis, you may be more motivated to make healthier choices.

3. Identifying triggers: Tracking your food intake can help you identify triggers for overeating or unhealthy eating habits. For example, you may notice that you tend to snack more in the afternoon or eat larger portions at dinner.

4. Personalization: By tracking your food intake, you can personalize your diet to meet your individual needs and goals. You can identify areas where you may be lacking in certain nutrients and make changes to address those gaps.

Conclusion

Keeping a food diary or using a food tracking app can be an effective way to monitor your food intake and promote weight loss. By becoming more aware of what you're eating and drinking, you can make changes to improve your diet and reach your weight loss goals. Remember to be consistent and honest with yourself when tracking your food intake, and use the information you gather to make positive changes in your diet and lifestyle.

Chapter 7: Mindful Eating Techniques to Prevent Overeating and Emotional Eating

Mindful eating is a practice that can help you develop a healthier relationship with food. It involves paying attention to your food and the act of eating, and being aware of your thoughts and feelings while you eat.

Here are some mindful eating techniques you can try to prevent overeating and emotional eating:

1. Slow down: Eating slowly can help you pay more attention to your food and become more aware of when you're full. Try putting your fork down between bites, and chew your food slowly and thoroughly.

2. Focus on your senses: Pay attention to the flavors, textures, and smells of your food. Notice how your body feels as you eat. This can help you become more present in the moment and enjoy your food more fully.

3. Practice gratitude: Before you eat, take a moment to express gratitude for your food and the people and resources that made it possible. This can help you appreciate your food and develop a more positive relationship with eating.

4. Tune in to your hunger and fullness cues: Check in with your body throughout your meal to see how hungry or full you feel. Stop eating when you're comfortably full, even if there's food left on your plate.

5. Avoid distractions: Eating while distracted, such as while watching TV or scrolling through your phone, can lead to mindless eating and overeating. Try to eat in a calm and distraction-free environment.

6. Recognize emotional eating: Pay attention to your emotions and how they may be affecting your eating habits. If you notice that you're turning to food to cope with stress, anxiety, or other emotions, try to find other ways to manage those feelings.

7. Don't restrict yourself: Restricting certain foods or food groups can lead to feelings of deprivation and overeating. Instead, focus on including a variety of foods in your diet and practicing moderation.

Benefits of Mindful Eating

Practicing mindful eating can have many benefits for weight loss and overall health. Here are some of the main benefits:

1. Improved digestion: Eating slowly and mindfully can help improve digestion and reduce digestive discomfort.

2. Weight loss: By becoming more aware of your hunger and fullness cues, you may be able to prevent overeating and promote weight loss.

3. Reduced stress and anxiety: Mindful eating can help reduce stress and anxiety by promoting a sense of calm and relaxation during meals.

4. Improved food choices: By paying attention to your food choices and how they make you feel, you can make healthier and more satisfying choices.

Conclusion

Mindful eating is a powerful tool for preventing overeating and emotional eating. By becoming more aware of your food and the act of eating, you can develop a healthier relationship with food and promote weight loss. Try incorporating some of these mindful eating techniques into your meals and see how they can help you become more present and mindful while you eat. Remember, developing a healthy relationship with food is a journey, and it's important to be patient and compassionate with yourself along the way.

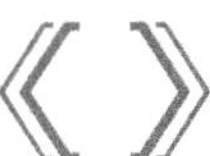

CHAPTER 8: DEVELOPING an Exercise Routine to Burn Calories and Increase Metabolism

In addition to following a healthy diet, exercise is an essential component of weight loss. Exercise can help you burn calories, increase your metabolism, and improve your overall health and fitness. Here are some tips for developing an exercise routine to support your weight loss goals:

1. Choose activities you enjoy: The key to sticking with an exercise routine is finding activities that you enjoy. Whether it's running, cycling, swimming, or dancing, find an activity that you look forward to and that fits into your schedule.

2. Set realistic goals: Start with small, achievable goals, and gradually increase the intensity and duration of your workouts as your fitness level improves. Setting realistic goals can help you stay motivated and avoid burnout.

3. Mix it up: Incorporate a variety of activities into your routine to keep things interesting and challenge your body in different ways. This can help prevent boredom

and plateaus in your progress.

4. Strength train: In addition to cardiovascular exercise, strength training is important for building muscle mass and boosting metabolism. Aim to include resistance training exercises, such as weight lifting or bodyweight exercises, two to three times per week.

5. Be consistent: Consistency is key when it comes to exercise. Aim to exercise at least 30 minutes per day, five days per week, or a total of 150 minutes per week.

6. Stay active throughout the day: In addition to formal exercise sessions, find ways to stay active throughout the day, such as taking the stairs instead of the elevator, going for a walk during your lunch break, or doing a quick workout video at home.

7. Get enough rest and recovery: Rest and recovery are important for preventing injuries and allowing your body to recover and rebuild after exercise. Aim for at least one rest day per week, and prioritize getting enough sleep and proper nutrition.

Benefits of Exercise for Weight Loss

Regular exercise has many benefits for weight loss and overall health. Here are some of the main benefits:

1. Burn calories: Exercise can help you burn calories and create a calorie deficit, which is necessary for weight loss.

2. Boost metabolism: Strength training can help increase muscle mass and boost metabolism, which can help you burn more calories throughout the day.

3. Reduce body fat: Exercise can help reduce body fat,

including visceral fat (the fat around your organs) which is linked to many health problems.

4. Improve cardiovascular health: Cardiovascular exercise can improve heart health and reduce the risk of chronic diseases, such as heart disease and diabetes.

5. Increase energy and stamina: Regular exercise can increase energy levels and improve physical performance, making it easier to perform daily activities and workouts.

Conclusion

Developing an exercise routine is an important part of weight loss and overall health. By choosing activities you enjoy, setting realistic goals, and being consistent, you can develop a sustainable exercise routine that supports your weight loss goals. Remember to also prioritize rest and recovery, and seek the guidance of a qualified fitness professional if you are new to exercise or have any health concerns. With regular exercise, you can boost your metabolism, burn calories, and improve your overall health and fitness.

Chapter 9: How to Create a Home Workout Routine Without Any Equipment

You don't need to have a gym membership or expensive equipment to get a great workout. With a little creativity, you can create a home workout routine that targets all of your major muscle groups and helps you burn calories and build strength. Here are some tips for creating a home workout routine without any equipment:

1. Warm up: Before starting any workout, it's important to warm up to prevent injuries and prepare your body for exercise. This can include dynamic stretching, jumping jacks, or a light cardio activity such as marching in place.

2. Focus on bodyweight exercises: Bodyweight exercises are exercises that use your own body weight as resistance. These can include exercises such as push-ups, squats, lunges, and planks. Bodyweight exercises are effective for building strength and can be modified to suit your fitness level.

3. Incorporate cardio: Cardiovascular exercise is important for burning calories and improving heart health. You can incorporate cardio into your home workout routine by doing exercises such as jumping jacks, high knees, or mountain climbers.

4. Use household items as weights: If you want to add resistance to your workout, you can use household items such as water bottles or cans of soup as weights. These items can be used for exercises such as bicep curls or shoulder presses.

5. Mix it up: To prevent boredom and challenge your body in different ways, mix up your exercises and routines. You can try different variations of bodyweight exercises or add new exercises to your routine.

6. Incorporate stretching and cool down: After your workout, it's important to stretch to improve flexibility and reduce muscle soreness. This can include static stretching or using a foam roller. Cooling down can also help your body recover and return to its resting state.

Sample Home Workout Routine:

Here's a sample home workout routine that you can do without any equipment:

Warm-up: 5-10 minutes of dynamic stretching, such as arm circles, high knees, and jumping jacks.

Circuit 1: Perform each exercise for 30 seconds, with 10 seconds of rest in between. Repeat the circuit three times.

- Squats
- Push-ups
- Plank
- Jumping jacks

Circuit 2: Perform each exercise for 30 seconds, with 10 seconds of rest in between. Repeat the circuit three times.

- Lunges
- Tricep dips (using a chair or bench)
- Bicycle crunches
- High knees

Cool down: 5-10 minutes of static stretching, focusing on the major muscle groups you worked during the workout.

Conclusion

Creating a home workout routine without any equipment is an effective way to stay active and improve your fitness without having to leave your home. By incorporating bodyweight exercises, cardio, and stretching, you can target all of your major muscle groups and burn calories. Remember to warm up, cool down, and modify exercises to suit your fitness level. With a little creativity, you can create a home workout routine that works for you and helps you reach your weight loss goals.

Chapter 10: Setting Realistic Weight Loss Goals and Tracking Progress

Setting realistic weight loss goals is important to ensure that you are making progress towards your desired weight and maintaining your motivation. However, it is also important to track your progress to know if you are on track and if any adjustments are needed. Here are some tips for setting realistic weight loss goals and tracking progress:

1. Determine your desired weight: The first step in setting a weight loss goal is determining your desired weight. It is important to be realistic and choose a weight that is healthy and attainable.

2. Break it down into smaller goals: Instead of setting one big goal, break it down into smaller goals. This will help you stay motivated and give you a sense of accomplishment as you reach each goal.

3. Make it measurable: Set a specific weight loss goal and make it measurable. For example, "I want to lose 1 pound per week for the next 10 weeks."

4. Use a tracking tool: Using a tracking tool, such as a weight loss journal or an app, can help you track your progress and stay motivated. This will also help you identify any patterns or areas where you may need to make adjustments.

5. Celebrate progress: Celebrate your progress along the way, even if it's small. This will help you stay motivated and focused on your goal.

6. Adjust as needed: If you are not making progress towards your goal, it may be time to re-evaluate and

make adjustments to your diet or exercise routine. It is important to be flexible and willing to adjust your approach as needed.

7. Don't focus on the number on the scale: While weight is an important factor in weight loss, it is not the only indicator of progress. Pay attention to how you feel, how your clothes fit, and other non-scale victories.

Conclusion

Setting realistic weight loss goals and tracking progress is important for achieving and maintaining weight loss. By breaking down your goal into smaller, measurable goals and using a tracking tool, you can stay motivated and make adjustments as needed. Celebrating progress along the way and focusing on non-scale victories can also help keep you motivated and focused on your goal. Remember to be flexible and willing to adjust your approach as needed to ensure success.

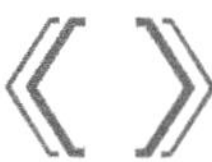

CHAPTER 11: STRATEGIES for Staying Motivated and Accountable

Losing weight can be a challenging journey, and it is important to stay motivated and accountable to achieve your goals. Here are some strategies that can help you stay motivated and accountable:

1. Set specific and realistic goals: Set specific and realistic weight loss goals that you can achieve. This will help you stay motivated and focused on your progress.

2. Find a support system: Having a support system can

help you stay motivated and accountable. This can be a friend, family member, or a support group.

3. Reward yourself: Rewarding yourself for achieving small goals can help you stay motivated. This can be a small treat or something that makes you feel good.

4. Visualize your success: Visualize yourself achieving your weight loss goals. This can help you stay motivated and focused on your progress.

5. Use positive self-talk: Use positive self-talk to keep yourself motivated. This can be affirmations or positive statements that help you stay focused on your goals.

6. Track your progress: Tracking your progress can help you stay accountable and motivated. This can be done through a weight loss journal or an app.

7. Be consistent: Consistency is key when it comes to weight loss. Stick to your meal plan, exercise routine, and self-care practices to see results.

8. Stay flexible: Be open to making changes to your routine and adjusting your goals as needed. This will help you stay motivated and avoid burnout.

9. Focus on the benefits: Focus on the benefits of weight loss, such as improved health, increased energy, and improved confidence.

10. Find joy in the journey: Find joy in the process of losing weight. Enjoy healthy meals, try new workouts, and find fun activities that support your goals.

Conclusion

Staying motivated and accountable is important for achieving and maintaining weight loss. By setting specific and realistic goals, finding a support system, rewarding yourself, visualizing success, using positive self-talk, tracking progress, being consistent, staying flexible, focusing on the benefits, and finding joy in the journey, you can stay motivated and accountable on your weight loss journey. Remember to be patient and kind to yourself, and celebrate every small victory along the way.

Chapter 12: Addressing Barriers to Weight Loss, such as Stress or Lack of Time

Losing weight can be challenging, and there are many barriers that can make it difficult to achieve and maintain weight loss. Here are some strategies for addressing common barriers to weight loss:

1. Stress: Stress can lead to overeating or emotional eating, which can make weight loss difficult. To address stress, consider practicing stress-reducing techniques such as meditation, yoga, or deep breathing exercises. It is also important to prioritize self-care practices such as getting enough sleep, staying hydrated, and engaging in activities that bring you joy.

2. Lack of time: Many people struggle to find the time to exercise or prepare healthy meals. To address this barrier, consider finding ways to incorporate physical activity into your daily routine, such as taking the stairs instead of the elevator, walking or biking to work, or finding a workout partner. Meal prep can also save time by preparing healthy meals in advance.

3. Lack of knowledge: Lack of knowledge about nutrition or exercise can make weight loss difficult. To address this barrier, consider working with a registered dietitian or personal trainer who can provide guidance and support.

4. Social situations: Social situations such as parties or dinners out can make it difficult to stick to a healthy diet. To address this barrier, consider planning ahead by bringing a healthy dish to share or looking at the

menu in advance to make healthier choices.

5. Plateaus: Plateaus can be discouraging and make it difficult to stay motivated. To address this barrier, consider adjusting your meal plan or exercise routine, or seeking support from a friend or professional.

6. Medical conditions: Medical conditions such as hypothyroidism or PCOS can make weight loss more challenging. To address this barrier, consult with your healthcare provider who can provide guidance and support.

Conclusion

There are many barriers to weight loss, but by addressing them with strategies such as stress reduction techniques, time management, seeking knowledge, planning ahead for social situations, overcoming plateaus, and consulting with healthcare providers for medical conditions, you can overcome these obstacles and achieve your weight loss goals. Remember to be patient and kind to yourself, and celebrate every small victory along the way.

Chapter 13: The Role of Sleep in Weight Loss and Strategies for Improving Sleep Quality

Sleep is an essential aspect of overall health and wellbeing, and it plays an important role in weight loss. Here are some ways that sleep affects weight loss and strategies for improving sleep quality:

How Sleep Affects Weight Loss

1. Hormonal changes: Lack of sleep can lead to hormonal changes that affect weight loss. Specifically, lack of sleep can increase levels of the hormone ghrelin, which stimulates appetite, and decrease levels of the hormone leptin, which signals fullness. This hormonal imbalance can lead to overeating and weight gain.
2. Metabolism: Sleep is essential for maintaining a healthy metabolism. Lack of sleep can slow down metabolism, making it harder to burn calories and lose weight.
3. Energy levels: Lack of sleep can lead to decreased energy levels, which can make it harder to stay motivated to exercise or prepare healthy meals.

Strategies for Improving Sleep Quality

1. Stick to a sleep schedule: Going to bed and waking up at the same time each day can help regulate your body's sleep-wake cycle and improve sleep quality.
2. Create a sleep-conducive environment: Make sure your bedroom is quiet, cool, and dark, and avoid using electronic devices in the bedroom.
3. Limit caffeine and alcohol intake: Caffeine and alcohol

can interfere with sleep quality, so it's important to limit intake, especially in the evening.

4. Practice relaxation techniques: Relaxation techniques such as deep breathing, meditation, or yoga can help reduce stress and promote better sleep.

5. Avoid large meals before bed: Eating a large meal before bed can make it harder to fall asleep and may cause indigestion.

6. Exercise regularly: Regular exercise can improve sleep quality and promote weight loss.

Conclusion

Sleep plays an important role in weight loss, and lack of sleep can make weight loss more difficult. By following strategies such as sticking to a sleep schedule, creating a sleep-conducive environment, limiting caffeine and alcohol intake, practicing relaxation techniques, avoiding large meals before bed, and exercising regularly, you can improve sleep quality and support your weight loss efforts. Remember, weight loss is a journey that requires patience, commitment, and a holistic approach to health and wellbeing.

Chapter 14: Tips for Dining Out and Making Healthier Choices at Restaurants

Eating out at restaurants can be a challenge when trying to lose weight, but it doesn't have to derail your progress. Here are some tips for making healthier choices when dining out:

1. Look up the menu beforehand: Most restaurants have their menus available online, so take a look before you go. This can help you plan ahead and choose healthier options.

2. Choose grilled or baked options: Instead of fried or breaded options, choose dishes that are grilled, baked, or roasted. These cooking methods are typically healthier and lower in calories.

3. Avoid creamy or cheesy sauces: Creamy or cheesy sauces can be high in calories and fat, so try to avoid them. Opt for tomato-based sauces or ask for dressing or sauce on the side.

4. Watch portion sizes: Restaurant portion sizes are often larger than what you would normally eat at home. Consider sharing an entrée with a friend or taking half of your meal home for leftovers.

5. Ask for modifications: Don't be afraid to ask for modifications to a dish. Ask for salad dressing on the side, skip the croutons or cheese, or ask for extra vegetables instead of a starch.

6. Choose healthier sides: Instead of fries or chips, choose healthier sides such as a side salad, steamed vegetables, or a baked sweet potato.

7. Practice mindful eating: Take your time eating and

enjoy each bite. Listen to your body's hunger and fullness signals and stop eating when you're satisfied.

8. Limit alcohol intake: Alcohol is high in calories and can also lower your inhibitions, making it harder to make healthy choices. Limit your alcohol intake or choose lower calorie options such as a glass of wine or a light beer.

9. Don't be too hard on yourself: Remember that dining out is meant to be enjoyable, so don't be too hard on yourself if you indulge in a less healthy option. The key is to balance your choices and make healthier choices most of the time.

Conclusion

Dining out at restaurants can be a challenge when trying to lose weight, but by following these tips and making healthier choices, you can still enjoy eating out while supporting your weight loss goals. Remember to plan ahead, choose grilled or baked options, watch portion sizes, ask for modifications, choose healthier sides, practice mindful eating, limit alcohol intake, and don't be too hard on yourself. With a little planning and mindfulness, you can make healthier choices while still enjoying dining out.

Chapter 15: Understanding Portion Control and How to Estimate Serving Sizes

Portion control is an important aspect of weight loss, as it can be easy to overeat and consume more calories than your body needs. Understanding portion sizes and how to estimate them can help you make healthier choices and manage your calorie intake. Here are some tips for understanding portion control and estimating serving sizes:

1. Use measuring tools: Using measuring cups, spoons, and a food scale can help you accurately measure serving sizes. This can be especially helpful when first learning about portion control.

2. Use visual cues: Visual cues can also be helpful in estimating serving sizes. For example, a serving of meat should be about the size of a deck of cards, a serving of pasta should be about the size of a tennis ball, and a serving of cheese should be about the size of a pair of dice.

3. Read labels: Pay attention to serving sizes on food labels, as they can be deceiving. For example, a package of crackers may list a serving size as only a few crackers, but you may end up eating the entire package, which can add up in calories.

4. Practice mindful eating: Mindful eating can also help with portion control. Slow down and pay attention to your hunger and fullness cues. Take breaks during your meal to assess whether you are still hungry or full.

5. Use smaller plates: Using smaller plates can also help with portion control by tricking your brain into

thinking you are eating more than you actually are.

6. Plan ahead: Planning your meals and snacks ahead of time can also help with portion control. Pre-portioning your meals and snacks can help you avoid overeating and make healthier choices.

7. Be aware of high calorie foods: Be mindful of foods that are high in calories and fat, such as fried foods, creamy sauces, and sugary drinks. These foods should be consumed in moderation or avoided altogether.

8. Listen to your body: Remember to listen to your body and stop eating when you are full. It is important to not feel obligated to finish your plate, especially when eating out.

Conclusion

Understanding portion control and estimating serving sizes can help with weight loss and overall healthy eating habits. Using measuring tools, visual cues, reading labels, practicing mindful eating, using smaller plates, planning ahead, being aware of high calorie foods, and listening to your body can all contribute to better portion control. By practicing portion control and making healthier choices, you can manage your calorie intake and support your weight loss goals.

Chapter 16: Strategies for Managing Cravings and Avoiding Temptation

Cravings can be a significant barrier to weight loss, as they can derail your healthy eating habits and lead to overeating. However, there are strategies you can use to manage cravings and avoid temptation. Here are some tips for managing cravings and avoiding temptation:

1. Identify triggers: Identify the triggers that lead to your cravings. Common triggers include stress, boredom, social situations, and certain foods. Once you identify your triggers, you can develop strategies to manage them.
2. Distract yourself: When you experience a craving, try distracting yourself with a non-food activity, such as going for a walk, calling a friend, or doing a puzzle.
3. Practice mindfulness: Mindfulness can also help with managing cravings. Pay attention to your thoughts and emotions when experiencing a craving, and try to be present in the moment.
4. Plan ahead: Planning ahead can help you avoid temptation. Prepare healthy snacks and meals ahead of time, and avoid keeping unhealthy foods in your home.
5. Use substitution: If you are craving a specific food, try finding a healthier substitute. For example, if you are craving something sweet, try eating fruit or a small piece of dark chocolate.
6. Allow for moderation: It is important to allow for moderation and enjoy occasional treats. Completely depriving yourself of your favorite foods can lead to binge eating and feeling deprived.
7. Get enough sleep: Lack of sleep can contribute to cravings, so make sure to prioritize getting enough sleep each night.
8. Seek support: Surround yourself with a supportive network of friends and family who can help you stay accountable and motivated.

Conclusion

Managing cravings and avoiding temptation is an important aspect of weight loss. Identifying triggers, distracting yourself, practicing mindfulness, planning ahead, using substitution, allowing for moderation, getting enough sleep, and seeking support can all help with managing cravings and avoiding temptation. By using these strategies, you can stay on track with your weight loss goals and develop healthier eating habits. Remember to be patient with yourself and allow for occasional treats, as long as they are consumed in moderation.

Chapter 17: Healthy Snacks to Keep on Hand for Weight Loss

Snacking can be an important part of a healthy diet, as it can help you manage hunger and prevent overeating at meals. However, it is important to choose healthy snacks that are low in calories and high in nutrients. Here are some healthy snacks to keep on hand for weight loss:

1. Fresh fruits: Fresh fruits are a great snack option, as they are low in calories and high in fiber and nutrients. Some great options include apples, bananas, berries, and grapes.
2. Vegetables and hummus: Raw vegetables, such as carrots, celery, and bell peppers, paired with hummus or another healthy dip, can make a satisfying and nutritious snack.
3. Greek yogurt: Greek yogurt is high in protein and low in calories, making it a great snack option. Add some fresh fruit or nuts for added flavor and nutrients.
4. Nuts and seeds: Nuts and seeds are a great source of healthy fats, fiber, and protein. Some good options include almonds, walnuts, cashews, and sunflower seeds.
5. Hard-boiled eggs: Hard-boiled eggs are a convenient and healthy snack option, as they are high in protein and low in calories.
6. Rice cakes and nut butter: Rice cakes paired with a healthy nut butter, such as almond or peanut butter, can make a satisfying and nutritious snack.
7. Air-popped popcorn: Air-popped popcorn is a low-

calorie snack option that can help satisfy cravings for something crunchy.

8. Cottage cheese and fruit: Cottage cheese paired with fresh fruit is a high-protein, low-calorie snack that can help keep you feeling full and satisfied.

9. Roasted chickpeas: Roasted chickpeas are a crunchy, high-protein snack option that can help satisfy cravings for something savory.

10. Smoothies: Smoothies made with fresh fruits and vegetables, Greek yogurt, and/or protein powder can make a nutritious and filling snack.

Conclusion

Snacking can be an important part of a healthy diet, but it is important to choose healthy snacks that are low in calories and high in nutrients. Fresh fruits, vegetables and hummus, Greek yogurt, nuts and seeds, hard-boiled eggs, rice cakes and nut butter, air-popped popcorn, cottage cheese and fruit, roasted chickpeas, and smoothies are all great snack options for weight loss. By keeping these healthy snacks on hand, you can manage hunger and prevent overeating at meals while still meeting your weight loss goals.

Chapter 18: The Role of Hydration in Weight Loss and How to Drink More Water

Drinking enough water is crucial for overall health and well-being, but it can also play an important role in weight loss. Here's why:

1. Water helps to increase metabolism: Drinking water can increase the number of calories your body burns at rest. This is because water helps to increase your metabolism, or the rate at which your body burns calories.

2. Water helps to reduce appetite: Drinking water before meals can help to reduce appetite and calorie intake. This is because water can help to fill your stomach, reducing the amount of food you consume.

3. Water helps to reduce fluid retention: When you are dehydrated, your body tends to retain fluid, which can lead to bloating and water weight gain. Drinking enough water can help to reduce fluid retention and promote weight loss.

So how much water should you be drinking? The amount of water you need can vary based on factors such as your age, gender, weight, and activity level. As a general rule, it is recommended to aim for at least 8 cups (64 ounces) of water per day.

Here are some tips for drinking more water:

1. Carry a water bottle with you: Having a water bottle with you at all times can help to remind you to drink more water throughout the day.

2. Flavor your water: If you find plain water boring, try adding some flavor to it. You can add sliced fruit, such as lemon or cucumber, or even a splash of fruit juice to your water to make it more appealing.
3. Drink water before meals: Drinking water before meals can help to reduce appetite and calorie intake.
4. Set reminders: Set reminders on your phone or computer to remind you to drink water throughout the day.
5. Eat water-rich foods: Eating foods that are high in water content, such as fruits and vegetables, can also help to increase your overall water intake.

Conclusion

Drinking enough water is important for overall health and well-being, but it can also play an important role in weight loss. Drinking water can help to increase metabolism, reduce appetite, and reduce fluid retention. Aim for at least 8 cups (64 ounces) of water per day and try carrying a water bottle with you, flavoring your water, drinking water before meals, setting reminders, and eating water-rich foods to help increase your water intake. By staying hydrated, you can promote weight loss and improve your overall health.

Chapter 19: Incorporating More Physical Activity into Your Daily Routine

In addition to a healthy diet, incorporating physical activity into your daily routine is essential for successful weight loss. Exercise helps to burn calories, increase metabolism, and improve overall health. Here are some tips for incorporating more physical activity into your daily routine:

1. Start small: If you are new to exercise, start with small goals and gradually increase the intensity and duration of your workouts. You can begin with a 10-minute walk and gradually work your way up to longer walks or runs.

2. Find an activity you enjoy: Choose an activity that you enjoy, such as swimming, dancing, or biking. When you enjoy the activity, you are more likely to stick with it and make it a part of your daily routine.

3. Schedule your workouts: Set aside time in your schedule for exercise and treat it like an important appointment. This can help you stay committed to your exercise routine.

4. Incorporate physical activity into your daily routine: Look for opportunities to incorporate physical activity into your daily routine. This can include taking the stairs instead of the elevator, walking to work or to run errands, or doing household chores that require physical activity.

5. Use technology to track your progress: Use a fitness tracker or smartphone app to track your steps, distance, and calories burned. This can help you stay

motivated and track your progress over time.

6. Mix it up: Vary your workouts to prevent boredom and challenge your body in new ways. You can try different types of exercise, such as yoga, strength training, or high-intensity interval training (HIIT).

7. Get support: Join a fitness class, hire a personal trainer, or find a workout buddy to provide support and accountability.

Conclusion

Incorporating physical activity into your daily routine is essential for successful weight loss. Start small, find an activity you enjoy, schedule your workouts, incorporate physical activity into your daily routine, use technology to track your progress, mix it up, and get support to stay motivated and on track. By making physical activity a part of your daily routine, you can burn calories, increase metabolism, and improve your overall health.

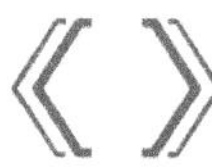

CHAPTER 20: CELEBRATING Milestones and Practicing Self-Compassion throughout the Weight Loss Journey

Losing weight is a journey that takes time, effort, and commitment. It is important to celebrate milestones along the way and practice self-compassion to stay motivated and positive. Here are some tips for celebrating milestones and practicing self-compassion throughout the weight loss journey:

1. Set realistic goals: Setting realistic goals can help you feel accomplished and motivated. Celebrate

milestones, such as losing a certain amount of weight or fitting into a smaller clothing size.

2. Find non-food rewards: Instead of using food as a reward, find non-food rewards that align with your goals, such as buying new workout gear, getting a massage, or taking a vacation.

3. Practice positive self-talk: Replace negative self-talk with positive affirmations. Focus on your progress and what you have accomplished, rather than your perceived shortcomings.

4. Embrace slip-ups as opportunities for growth: Slip-ups are a natural part of the weight loss journey. Instead of beating yourself up over a mistake, view it as an opportunity to learn and grow. Reflect on what caused the slip-up and come up with a plan to prevent it from happening again in the future.

5. Practice self-care: Practicing self-care can help reduce stress and improve overall well-being. This can include activities such as taking a bubble bath, practicing yoga, or getting enough sleep.

6. Seek support: Surround yourself with supportive friends and family who encourage and motivate you. Join a support group or seek out professional help if needed.

7. Remember the bigger picture: Remember that weight loss is not just about looking better, but also about improving your overall health and well-being. Celebrate the progress you have made and remember the positive impact it will have on your life.

Conclusion

Celebrating milestones and practicing self-compassion throughout the weight loss journey is essential for long-term success. Set realistic goals, find non-food rewards, practice positive self-talk, embrace slip-ups as opportunities for growth, practice self-care, seek support, and remember the bigger picture. By celebrating your accomplishments and practicing self-compassion, you can stay motivated and positive throughout the weight loss journey.

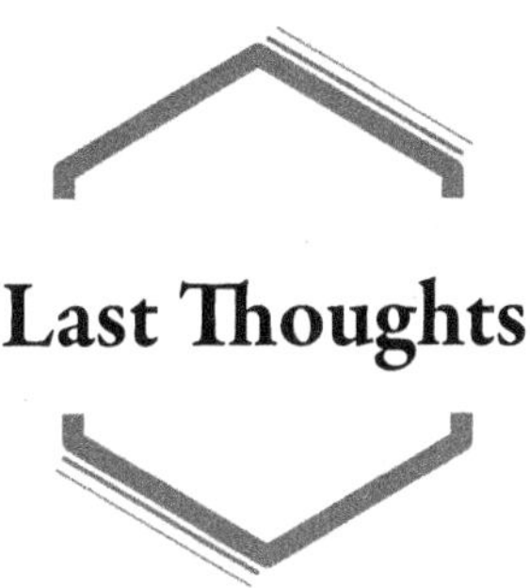

Last Thoughts

As I sit down to write these final thoughts on my weight loss journey, a rush of emotions and memories floods my mind. It's hard to believe that this transformative journey, which consumed so much of my life, is coming to an end. But as I reflect on the past months and years, I realize that the end of this chapter marks the beginning of a new and empowered chapter in my life.

Weight loss is a deeply personal and multifaceted journey. It's not just about shedding physical pounds; it's about shedding self-doubt, limiting beliefs, and the emotional baggage that often accompanies excess weight. Throughout my own experience, I've come to understand that true and lasting weight loss extends beyond the physical realm—it encompasses a holistic transformation of mind, body, and spirit.

One of the most crucial lessons I've learned on this journey is the importance of self-compassion. It's all too easy to fall into the trap of self-criticism and negative self-talk, especially when progress seems slow or setbacks occur. But berating ourselves only perpetuates the cycle of self-sabotage. Instead, I've discovered the power of treating myself with kindness, understanding, and forgiveness. Embracing self-compassion has allowed me to celebrate my victories, no matter how small, and to approach setbacks as opportunities for growth rather than reasons to give up.

Another key aspect of successful weight loss is cultivating a healthy relationship with food. For far too long, food was my source of comfort, my solace in times of stress or emotional turmoil. But through this journey, I've learned to view food as nourishment for both my body and soul. I've discovered the joy of mindful eating, savoring each bite, and appreciating the nourishing qualities of wholesome foods. It's not about deprivation or rigid rules; it's about making conscious choices that honor my body's needs and fuel my overall well-being. Additionally, surrounding myself with a support network has been instrumental in my success. Weight loss can feel isolating at times, and having a community of like-minded individuals who understand the challenges and triumphs is invaluable. Whether it's friends, family, or online communities, having people who cheer you on, provide guidance, and offer a listening ear can make all the difference. We're not meant to walk this journey alone, and by reaching out for support, we gain strength and resilience.

Perhaps one of the most profound realizations I've had is that weight loss is not a destination; it's a lifelong journey. Maintaining a healthy weight requires ongoing commitment, self-awareness, and adaptability. I've come to understand that the number on the scale is not the sole measure of success. It's about prioritizing my well-being, embracing a balanced lifestyle, and nurturing a positive body image. I refuse to let my worth be defined by a number; instead, I focus on cultivating self-love, self-acceptance, and gratitude for the incredible vessel that is my body.

As I conclude this chapter, I want to extend my deepest gratitude to all those who have supported me along the way. To my loved ones who cheered me on and believed in me even when I doubted myself, thank you for your unwavering support. To the countless individuals who shared their own stories and offered guidance, thank you for inspiring me and reminding me that I am not alone.

To anyone who may be embarking on their own weight loss journey, I offer you these parting words of encouragement. Believe in yourself, for you are capable of more than you can imagine. Embrace the process, for it is in the journey that you will discover your true strength. And above all, love yourself fiercely and unconditionally, for you are deserving of a life of joy, vitality, and self-fulfillment.

Remember that this journey is not just about reaching a certain number on the scale; it's about reclaiming your health, your confidence, and your zest for life. Embrace the small victories along the way—the increased energy, the improved sleep, the clothing sizes that start to shrink. These are the tangible reminders that you are making progress, even when the scale may not reflect it.

Stay curious and open-minded throughout your journey. Explore different approaches to nutrition and exercise, and find what works best for you. There is no one-size-fits-all solution when it comes to weight loss. Listen to your body, pay attention to how different foods make you feel, and find activities that bring you joy and make you want to move. This is not a punishment; it's an opportunity to discover the boundless potential within you.

Remember that setbacks are not signs of failure; they are stepping stones to growth. There will be days when you may indulge a little too much or skip a workout. That's okay. Be kind to yourself, acknowledge the slip-up, and use it as a learning experience. The key is to pick yourself up and keep moving forward. Progress is not linear, but as long as you stay committed to your goals and maintain a positive mindset, you will continue to make strides towards a healthier you. Celebrate your non-scale victories along the way. Notice how your confidence grows, how your clothes fit better, and how your overall well-being improves. Take pride in the small lifestyle changes you've made—the healthier meal choices, the consistent exercise routine, the moments of self-care. These seemingly insignificant actions add up to create a foundation for lasting change.

As you continue on this journey, remember that self-love and self-acceptance are paramount. Your worth is not determined by a number on the scale or the opinions of others. Embrace your unique beauty, both inside and out. Treat yourself with kindness, compassion, and respect. Surround yourself with positive influences and affirmations that uplift and inspire you. Remember that you are deserving of love, happiness, and good health at every stage of your journey.

In closing, know that you are not alone. Countless individuals around the world are on their own weight loss journeys, each with their own struggles and triumphs. Connect with others, share your story, and draw strength from the collective support and encouragement. Together, we can uplift and empower one another.

As I bid farewell to this chapter of my life, I do so with immense gratitude for the lessons learned, the strength gained, and the person I have become. My hope is that my journey and the insights shared within this book have provided guidance, inspiration, and motivation to all who read it.

May you embark on your weight loss journey with unwavering determination, self-compassion, and a belief in your own power to transform. Remember, you have the ability to drop those pounds, embrace a healthier lifestyle, and create the life you've always envisioned.

Wishing you a future filled with abundant health, joy, and fulfillment.

With heartfelt sincerity,

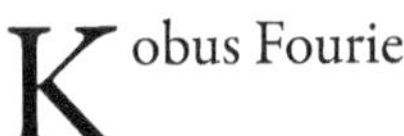
Kobus Fourie

Apps to help you on your journey:

There are numerous apps available that can help you track your weight loss progress. Here are some popular ones:

1. MyFitnessPal: MyFitnessPal is a free app that allows you to track your calorie intake and exercise. You can set weight loss goals and track your progress over time.

2. Lose It!: Lose It! is a free app that helps you set weight loss goals and track your progress. You can track your food intake, exercise, and connect with friends for accountability and support.

3. Noom: Noom is a paid app that offers personalized coaching and support for weight loss. It includes a food diary, exercise tracker, and educational resources to help you make healthy lifestyle changes.

4. Weight Watchers: Weight Watchers is a paid app that offers a point-based system for tracking food intake. It also includes personalized coaching and support.

5. Happy Scale: Happy Scale is a free app that helps you track your weight loss progress over time. It uses a trend line to show your overall progress, rather than focusing on daily fluctuations.

6. Fitbit: Fitbit is a fitness tracking app that also includes a weight loss tracker. You can track your food intake, exercise, and weight loss progress all in one place.

7. Fooducate: Fooducate is a free app that helps you make healthier food choices. It includes a barcode scanner to help you easily track the nutritional value of the foods you eat.

Remember that while apps can be helpful tools in tracking weight loss progress, they should not replace the advice and support of a healthcare professional. It is important to talk to your doctor before starting any weight loss program, and to seek professional help if you are struggling to lose weight.

ABOUT THE AUTHOR

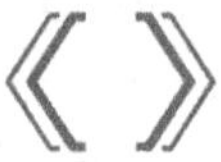

KOBUS FOURIE IS A WRITER with a passion for health and wellness. While he is not a certified expert in weight loss, he has a wealth of personal experience in the field. After struggling with his weight for many years, Kobus decided to take charge of his health and embarked on a journey to lose over 40 kilograms. Along the way, he learned valuable lessons about the challenges of weight loss, as well as effective strategies for achieving sustainable, long-term results.

In this book, Kobus shares his knowledge and insights, as well as the stories of others who have successfully transformed their bodies and lives through weight loss. He hopes that this book will inspire and motivate readers to make positive changes in their own lives and achieve their weight loss goals.

Don't miss out!

Visit the website below and you can sign up to receive emails whenever Kobus Fourie publishes a new book. There's no charge and no obligation.

https://books2read.com/r/B-A-KVXX-YRNIC

BOOKS 2 READ

Connecting independent readers to independent writers.

Also by Kobus Fourie

Strange Facts and Wonders
20 Beddie Buy Stories For Kid's
Animals by the Alphabet
Stop That Bad Smoking Habit
Drop Those Extra Pounds
Lyric's For Everyone

www.ingramcontent.com/pod-product-compliance
Lightning Source LLC
Chambersburg PA
CBHW060911130726
48001CB00006B/2193